# HOW TO GUIDE: CIALIS

A concise Handbook on how to use Cialis oral tablet to treat erectile dysfunction (ED) and benign prostatic hyperplasia (BPH)

**Dr. Diana Peters**

# Table of Contents

## OVERVIEW OF ERECTILE DYSFUNCTION

Erectile dysfunction (ED) is a common medical condition characterized by the inability to achieve or maintain an erection sufficient for satisfactory sexual performance. This condition affects millions of men worldwide and can have profound psychological, emotional, and relational impacts. ED can result from various factors, including cardiovascular diseases, diabetes, hormonal imbalances, neurological disorders, and psychological issues such as stress, anxiety, or depression. Lifestyle factors such as smoking, alcohol consumption, and lack of physical activity can also contribute to the development of ED.

### History and Development of Cialis

Cialis, known generically as tadalafil, is one of the most widely used medications for the treatment of erectile dysfunction. It was developed by the pharmaceutical company Eli Lilly in collaboration with ICOS Corporation. The development of Cialis was part of a broader effort to create a new class of ED medications known as phosphodiesterase type 5 (PDE5) inhibitors. Cialis was approved by the U.S. Food and Drug Administration (FDA) in 2003 and has since become a popular choice for men seeking treatment for ED.

The discovery of PDE5 inhibitors dates back to the early 1990s when scientists were researching treatments for cardiovascular diseases. During these studies, it was found that PDE5 inhibitors could enhance blood flow to specific areas of the body, including the penis. This led to the development of the first ED medication, sildenafil (Viagra), followed by vardenafil (Levitra) and tadalafil (Cialis). Each of these medications has unique properties, but Cialis is particularly noted for its longer duration of action.

## How Cialis Works

Cialis works by inhibiting the action of the enzyme phosphodiesterase type 5 (PDE5). PDE5 is primarily responsible for the breakdown of cyclic guanosine monophosphate (cGMP), a molecule that promotes the relaxation of smooth muscle tissues and increases blood flow to the penis during sexual stimulation. By inhibiting PDE5, Cialis helps to maintain higher levels of cGMP, leading to prolonged smooth muscle relaxation and improved blood flow to the penis, which facilitates an erection.

Unlike some other ED medications that have a shorter duration of action, Cialis is known for its prolonged effectiveness. It can remain active in the body for up to 36 hours, earning it the nickname "the weekend pill." This extended window of effectiveness allows for greater spontaneity in sexual activities, as men do not need to time the medication as precisely as they would with other treatments.

In summary, the introduction to Cialis encompasses a comprehensive understanding of erectile dysfunction, the historical development and approval of the medication, and its mechanism of action. This section provides readers with a foundational knowledge of Cialis, setting the stage for more detailed discussions on its usage, benefits, and considerations in the chapters that follow.

## ACTIVE INGREDIENTS AND THEIR EFFECTS

Cialis is primarily composed of tadalafil, the active ingredient responsible for its therapeutic effects. Tadalafil belongs to a class of drugs known as phosphodiesterase type 5 (PDE5) inhibitors. PDE5 inhibitors work by blocking the action of the enzyme PDE5, which breaks down cyclic guanosine monophosphate (cGMP). By inhibiting PDE5, tadalafil helps maintain higher levels of cGMP, leading to prolonged smooth muscle relaxation and increased blood flow to the penis during sexual stimulation. This enhanced blood flow facilitates the achievement and maintenance of an erection.

In addition to tadalafil, Cialis tablets contain inactive ingredients that serve as fillers, binders, and preservatives to ensure the stability and efficacy of the medication. These inactive ingredients do not contribute to the therapeutic effects but are essential for the overall formulation of the tablet.

## How Cialis Differs from Other ED Medications

Cialis is one of several medications available for the treatment of erectile dysfunction. It is often compared to other PDE5 inhibitors, such as sildenafil (Viagra) and vardenafil (Levitra). While all three medications share a similar mechanism of action, there are key differences that make Cialis unique:

- **Duration of Action**: Cialis is known for its long duration of action, which can last up to 36 hours. This extended effectiveness allows for greater spontaneity in sexual activity, as men do not need to time the medication as precisely as with other ED treatments. In contrast, sildenafil and vardenafil typically have a shorter duration of action, lasting around 4 to 6 hours.

- **Onset of Action**: Cialis typically begins to work within 30 minutes to 2 hours after ingestion, which is comparable to the onset time of sildenafil and vardenafil. However, individual response times can vary.

- **Daily Use Option**: Cialis is available in a lower-dose formulation (2.5 mg and 5 mg) for daily use. This regimen is beneficial for men who anticipate frequent sexual activity (e.g., several times a week). Daily use of Cialis ensures that the medication is always in the system, allowing for more spontaneous sexual encounters without the need to plan ahead. This option is not available for sildenafil or vardenafil.

- **Food Interactions**: Unlike sildenafil and vardenafil, which can be affected by high-fat meals, Cialis can be taken with or without food without significantly impacting its effectiveness. This flexibility can make it more convenient for users.

## Benefits of Using Cialis

Cialis offers several benefits for men with erectile dysfunction:

- **Extended Duration**: The prolonged duration of action (up to 36 hours) allows for more spontaneous and natural sexual activity, reducing the pressure to time the medication precisely.

- **Flexible Dosing Options**: The availability of both as-needed and daily dosing regimens provides flexibility to suit individual needs and preferences.

- **Improved Quality of Life**: Effective treatment of ED with Cialis can enhance sexual satisfaction, improve self-esteem, and strengthen intimate relationships.

- **Efficacy**: Clinical studies have shown that Cialis is highly effective in improving erectile function in men with ED, with a favorable safety profile.

Understanding these aspects of Cialis helps users make informed decisions about their treatment options, ensuring they choose the medication that best fits their lifestyle and medical needs. The next chapter will delve into the practical aspects of using Cialis, including recommended dosages, administration guidelines, and what to expect during treatment.

## RECOMMENDED DOSAGES

Cialis is available in several dosages to cater to different needs and preferences:

- **As-Needed Dosage**: Cialis is commonly prescribed in 10 mg and 20 mg doses for use on an as-needed basis. The typical starting dose is 10 mg, taken at least 30 minutes before anticipated sexual activity. Depending on efficacy and tolerability, the dose may be increased to 20 mg or decreased to 5 mg. The maximum recommended frequency is once per day.

- **Daily Dosage**: For men who prefer regular medication to allow for more spontaneous sexual activity, Cialis is available in 2.5 mg and 5 mg doses for daily use. The recommended starting dose is 2.5 mg taken at the same time each day, without regard to the timing of sexual activity. If the 2.5 mg dose is not effective, it can be increased to 5 mg daily.

## How to Take Cialis Correctly

To maximize the effectiveness of Cialis and minimize potential side effects, follow these guidelines:

- **As-Needed Use**: Take Cialis at least 30 minutes before sexual activity. The medication can be effective for up to 36 hours, allowing for flexibility in timing.

- **Daily Use**: Take Cialis at the same time each day, with or without food. Consistent daily use ensures that the medication is always present in your system, providing continuous efficacy.

- **Avoid Exceeding the Recommended Dose**: Do not take more than the prescribed dose. Taking more than the recommended amount does not increase the effectiveness and may increase the risk of side effects.

- **Follow Your Healthcare Provider's Instructions**: Always adhere to the dosage and administration guidelines provided by your healthcare provider.

## Timing and Duration of Effectiveness

Cialis is known for its long duration of action, which can last up to 36 hours. This extended window of effectiveness allows men to engage in sexual activity at any point within this period without the need for precise timing. The onset of action for Cialis typically occurs within 30 minutes to 2 hours after ingestion. However, individual response times may vary based on factors such as age, overall health, and the presence of other medical conditions.

## What to Expect After Taking Cialis

After taking Cialis, most men can expect the following:

- **Improved Erectile Function**: Cialis helps achieve and maintain an erection sufficient for satisfactory sexual activity when sexually stimulated.

- **Long-Lasting Effects**: The effects of Cialis can last up to 36 hours, providing a prolonged period during which erections can be achieved with sexual stimulation.

- **Variable Onset Time**: While Cialis generally starts working within 30 minutes to 2 hours, the exact onset time may vary from person to person.

It is important to note that Cialis will not cause an erection without sexual stimulation. The medication enhances the natural erectile response to sexual arousal but does not initiate an erection on its own.

By understanding how to use Cialis correctly, men can maximize the benefits of the medication while minimizing potential risks and side effects. The next chapter will explore the relationship between Cialis and overall health, including potential side effects, interactions with other medications, and important safety considerations.

## POTENTIAL SIDE EFFECTS

Like all medications, Cialis can cause side effects. While many men who take Cialis experience no or mild side effects, it's important to be aware of potential reactions:

- **Common Side Effects**:

    - Headache

    - Indigestion or heartburn

    - Back pain

    - Muscle aches

    - Flushing (redness of the face, neck, or chest)

    - Nasal congestion

- **Less Common Side Effects**:

    - Dizziness

    - Blurred vision

- Changes in color vision

  - Ringing in the ears

- **Serious Side Effects** (rare, but require immediate medical attention):

  - An erection lasting more than four hours (priapism)

  - Sudden loss of vision in one or both eyes (a sign of a serious eye problem called non-arteritic anterior ischemic optic neuropathy, or NAION)

  - Sudden decrease or loss of hearing

## Interactions with Other Medications

Cialis can interact with various medications, which may enhance or diminish its effects or increase the risk of side effects. Important interactions to be aware of include:

- **Nitrates**: Taking Cialis with nitrates (medications prescribed for chest pain, such as nitroglycerin) can cause a severe drop in blood pressure, leading to dizziness, fainting, or even heart attack or stroke. This combination should be strictly avoided.

- **Alpha-Blockers**: Used to treat high blood pressure and prostate problems, alpha-blockers can also cause a significant drop in blood pressure when taken with Cialis. If combination therapy is necessary, it should be started with the lowest possible doses.

- **Antihypertensives**: Combining Cialis with blood pressure medications can enhance the blood pressure-lowering effect. Monitoring and dose adjustments may be needed.

- **CYP3A4 Inhibitors**: Medications such as ketoconazole, ritonavir, and erythromycin can increase the levels of Cialis in the blood, leading to an increased risk of side effects. Dose adjustments of Cialis may be required.

- **Alcohol**: Excessive alcohol consumption can increase the risk of side effects like dizziness, headache, and low blood pressure.

## Contraindications and Warnings

Certain individuals should not take Cialis or should use it with caution. Contraindications and warnings include:

- **Cardiovascular Conditions**: Men with significant heart disease, recent heart attack, stroke, or severe heart failure should avoid Cialis. Sexual activity may strain the heart, particularly in those with underlying cardiovascular issues.

- **Liver or Kidney Impairment**: Dosage adjustments may be necessary for men with liver or kidney problems. Severe impairment may contraindicate use.

- **Allergic Reactions**: Anyone with a known allergy to tadalafil or any of the inactive ingredients in Cialis should not take the medication.

- **Peyronie's Disease**: Men with this condition, characterized by curvature of the penis, should use Cialis cautiously, as it may exacerbate the condition.

## Managing Side Effects

Most side effects of Cialis are mild and temporary. Here are some tips for managing common side effects:

- **Headache**: Over-the-counter pain relievers like acetaminophen or ibuprofen can help alleviate headaches. Staying hydrated and resting may also be beneficial.

- **Indigestion**: Avoiding large or rich meals and eating smaller, more frequent meals can help reduce indigestion. Antacids may also provide relief.

- **Muscle Aches**: Warm baths, stretching exercises, and over-the-counter pain relievers can help ease muscle aches.

- **Flushing and Nasal Congestion**: These symptoms usually diminish as the body adjusts to the medication. Drinking cool fluids and using a humidifier can help alleviate discomfort.

By understanding the potential side effects and interactions of Cialis, as well as who should avoid its use, men can make informed decisions about their health. The next chapter will discuss the use of Cialis in special populations and considerations for those with specific health conditions.

conclusion

Cialis has proven to be a valuable and effective treatment for erectile dysfunction, offering men a reliable option to improve their sexual health and quality of life. By understanding the intricacies of Cialis, from its development and mechanism of action to its proper usage and potential health impacts, individuals can make informed decisions and maximize the benefits of this medication.

## Summary of Key Points

- **Understanding Erectile Dysfunction**: Recognizing the causes and impact of erectile dysfunction is essential for addressing the condition effectively. Cialis provides a solution by enhancing blood flow to the penis, facilitating erections in response to sexual stimulation.

- **Development and Mechanism**: The history and development of Cialis underscore its effectiveness and safety. As a PDE5 inhibitor, Cialis works by maintaining higher levels of cGMP, leading to prolonged smooth muscle relaxation and improved erectile function.

- **Proper Usage**: Adhering to recommended dosages and administration guidelines ensures optimal results. Whether taken on an as-needed basis or daily, Cialis offers flexibility to suit different lifestyles and needs.

- **Health Considerations**: Awareness of potential side effects, interactions with other medications, and contraindications is crucial for safe use. By consulting healthcare providers and managing side effects appropriately, users can minimize risks and enhance their experience with Cialis.

- **Special Populations**: Understanding how Cialis interacts with various health conditions and special populations ensures that the medication is used safely and effectively by all who need it.

## Final Thoughts and Encouragement

The journey to better sexual health and overall well-being often involves addressing sensitive and personal issues such as erectile dysfunction. Cialis offers a viable and effective solution for many men, empowering them to regain confidence and improve their intimate relationships. By staying informed and working closely with healthcare providers, users can navigate the complexities of erectile dysfunction treatment and achieve the desired outcomes.

As you move forward, remember that seeking help for erectile dysfunction is a positive step towards improving your health and quality of life. With the right information and support, you can make the best choices for your individual needs. Cialis is a powerful tool in this journey, offering hope and tangible benefits for those seeking to enhance their sexual health and overall well-being.

Thank you for reading this guide on Cialis. We hope it has provided valuable insights and practical advice to help you make informed decisions about your treatment options. If you have any further questions or concerns, do not hesitate to reach out to your healthcare provider for personalized guidance and support.

# THE END